Adult
Advanced Life Support
2010 - 2015
by
Jamie Bisson

(Dip. H.Sc., Dip. N.Sc., B.Sc. (Hons.) Crit. Care)

Table of Contents

<u>Dedication</u>

This book is dedicated to my darling wife, Jo, who without the endless support and patience I would not be half the person I am today. She has put up with the hours of solitude that I have endured to write the many books published so far and to her I am eternally grateful.

Thank you for being there and for being here now.

-x-

Foreword

People say, some things in life are inevitable...... taxes and death. Well I cannot help you with your taxes, but I can help with reducing the risk of death to some degree.

I have been working in critical care since 1998 and am an authorised instructor of advanced life support. I can therefore give you the right information in the right way for you to fully understand the principles of resuscitation that this book covers.

People in healthcare often have to care for very sick individuals and a cardiorespiratory arrest is a real risk for many in our care. Knowing how to care for the patient to prevent a cardiorespiratory arrest and help the patient recover from their ailment is every healthcare professionals goal, however sometimes all the best care and intentions in the world do not prevent the patient from arresting.

This book will give you the necessary knowledge to understand basic and advanced life support for when you gain the appropriate local accreditation and authorisation from a medical governing body. The information in this book is based upon the best level of evidence available today. Guidelines and the treatments discussed in this book are supported by ILCOR (International Liaison Committee on Resuscitation) and the many of the Resuscitation Councils worldwide.

This book will mainly focus upon adult basic and advanced life support, as paediatric life support needs specialised focus and it is outside of the scope of this book. In the immediate future I will release a book on paediatric basic and advanced life support.

In no way, whatsoever am I the author, responsible for any care, or omission of care, provided by you or anyone else upon reading this book. It is for information and reference only and to be fully competent an authorising and regulatory body must have performed an assessment on your competence. Even so, after their assessment of your competence you are responsible for the care you provide and any omissions. However it is important to understand that some life support knowledge is better than none at all!

Recognising An Emergency

Recognising an emergency is the first step in dealing effectively with any emergency[1]. This should be done quickly to reduce the potential time that the heart is not circulating oxygenated blood. If there are two victims, the unconscious victim takes priority over the other victim as assessments need to be made regarding their level of consciousness, their airway and their respiratory effort.

There are many causes for unconsciousness. Each cause is enough for the person to become unconscious, but on some occasions there are a couple of causes present for example an intoxicated person who suffers a head injury or seizure. The causes include:

• Neurological issues for example a stroke or traumatic brain injury, malignancy or seizure[2].

• Cardiac arrhythmias, or severely low blood pressure[2].

• Ingestion of a sedating substance such as an overdose, alcohol intoxication, hypoglycaemia, otherwise known as a low blood sugar level[2].

• Hypoxaemia or low oxygen levels in the blood, which cause the brain to suffer ischaemia and fainting may occur[2].

When an emergency has been recognised it is essential that the basic life support (BLS) algorithm shown later in this book be followed.

The general principles of care in an emergency are as follows:

• Prevent further harm or injury

- Check for response

- Airway and breathing care / support

- Control of any bleeding

- Protection from exposure from the weather

- First aid

- Handling the patient gently

- Continual reassurance

- Continual observation

Basic Life Support

BLS is a skill that should be taught to all health care professionals and is a very worthwhile skill for the lay person to have. It is basically the ability to support the cardio-respiratory system until some advanced life support can be provided by a healthcare professional. BLS training has been shown to increase the rates of bystander life support provision, whilst increasing the chance of survival[3].

The principle of "simplicity is best" is adopted by the BLS algorithm in an effort that the lay person can follow the procedure with ease.

It is also true that some attempt to provide life saving CPR is better than no attempt at all if the patient is suffering a cardiopulmonary arrest. Therefore the provision of CPR should not be discouraged at any point in the absence of any immovable danger to the provider. It is also true to acknowledge if the provider of CPR develops any chest pain or severe shortness of breath should stop to reduce the risk of them also requiring medical attention[4].

The Australian and the New Zealand Resuscitation Council have produced a simple flow chart that can easily be followed by anyone:

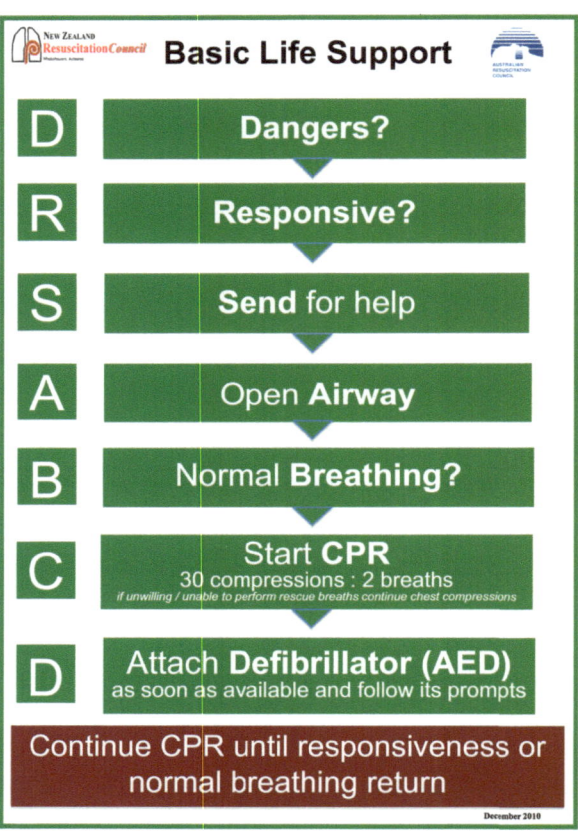

As can be seen the flow chart is broken into the simple mnemonic "DR'S ABCD" (without punctuation).

D: Danger

Danger and risk of danger must be managed in all situations. In the event of an emergency it is imperative to assess if it is safe for the rescuer to approach the victim. This will reduce the risk of the one victim becoming two. In addition to ensuring safety for the rescuer it is also important to ensure safety for any bystanders.

The victim may need to be moved in some circumstances, for example if they are lying in the middle of a road or railway. The victim will need to be moved if they are face down as to facilitate the assessment of their breathing and airway patency[5]. The concern of spinal injury should not stop the patient being moved should there be any concern that their airway was not clear or that they were not breathing normally. It is important to note that any patient with a suspected spinal injury who airway was not patent, should have a jaw-thrust manoeuvre performed prior to moving to attempt opening the airway. This manoeuvre will be discussed later. The rescuer needs to be aware and facilitate the safest possible way of moving the patient wherever possible. The avoidance of bending or twisting the victims neck is essential and if possible 3 - 5 people should be used to perform a "log-roll" where a concern of a spinal injury is present. A "log-roll" is a method of turning a person with the least twisting or bending of the entire spine. The rescuer needs to be aware that movement however may cause further clinical instability, pain, shock, blood loss and further injury. A risk to benefit ratio needs to be made to ensure safety for all. If a patient is breathing normally, then they should be left on their side in a recovery position.

With regards to a road traffic accident it is not safe to touch a vehicle, or rescue a victim from within the car within 10 meters of a fallen power line unless the electricity authority has deemed it safe to approach[6]. The use of bystanders to guide and warn traffic is essential to reduce the risk of further harm to both rescuer and victim. The use of hazard lights, triangles and torches will also be advantageous. When at the vehicle, attempt turning the ignition off and activating the hand or parking brake. If the parking brake is unaccessible then an option would be to place a block or rock under a wheel. It may be necessary to remove a motorbike from its rider. Wherever possible try to manage a breathing patient within the car without moving them unless there is a risk of harm or further injury by leaving them inside the vehicle[6].

In cases of electrocution it is essential not to touch the victim where the electric source is still live and within 10 meters of them[6]. If power lines are over a vehicle do not touch the victim or vehicle. Be aware of any water or other conductible debris and ensure that a 10 meter gap is present between you and the electricity source. Wherever possible disconnect the electricity, such as is possible within a home environment. Unplugging the device from the wall further reduces the risk of electric shock. BLS treatment should be performed when safe to do so and treatment of burns may also be necessary following an electrocution.

R: Response

Once the emergency has been identified and the risk of danger has been assessed and dealt with as necessary, it is important to gauge a sense of the victims response. Talk to the victim in a raised voice and touch them with some reasonable vigour by their shoulders or chest. In the case of a child or infant it is important to assess their response also, but often just a vigorous rub of their chest is enough to illicit a response if they are conscious. The idea of "shaking a baby" can give rise to some negative thoughts, but it is important to assess a child or infants response in the right manner and we are not suggesting that the child be picked up and shaken, but a talk and touch in the right manner, for example by the shoulders or a vigorous rub of the chest will often suffice.

It is important to be aware of any obvious injury and not shake that area where possible. If there is any concern of a spinal injury then the patient should not be shaken to such a degree that would cause spinal bending or twisting.

A raised voice when talking to the patient is important as the victim may have some hearing impairment and raising your voice is more likely to overcome this.

S: Send For Help

If the victim does not respond it is important to get help from trained personnel as soon as possible. If there are two rescuers present it is suggested that the person who is most experienced with resuscitation remain with the victim to potentially provide life saving interventions whilst the other person goes and gets help and a defibrillator if possible.

When an adult collapses it is most likely that they have suffered from a rhythm that can be treated with a defibrillator and as such the best way to get a positive outcome is to obtain a defibrillator as soon as possible. Defibrillators are often found in major public areas, such as malls, shopping precincts, supermarkets, airports, train / bus stations and in some cases churches.

The majority of time the way of getting help is by phoning for an ambulance or within a healthcare setting it is simply by asking for help and perhaps phoning for a rapid response team or activating a "code blue". In a public place there may be a defibrillator nearby so the experienced individual should take charge by stating their experience and staying with the individual and getting a bystander to get a nearby defibrillator whilst sending someone else to call an ambulance.

It is very important that if we are relying on an individual to get some help from trained personnel then they should be told to return and let us know that they have sought help and

that help is coming. If this is not done we may think that help has been called, when in fact it may not have been.

A: Airway

The airway of an unconscious person is easily obstructed by their tongue, which can flop onto the back of the throat completely blocking any air passage from the lungs. If this is left untreated asphyxiation and death will be the result. The same can happen with a foreign object or food/vomitus.

When foreign objects stimulate the vocal cords an innate reflex called laryngeal spasm occurs which is supposed to stop material, such as food, from continuing to the lungs. This may cause a temporary blockage of the airway and the patient may produce a bizarre noise from their throat called a stridor. A stridor can be heard by following this link http://www.rale.ca/media/stridor.wav. If the blockage is complete then no air will pass over the vocal cords and as such no noise will be produced, no air will move in or out of the lungs and the patient will be unable to breath at all. The patient will then go blue and become unconscious. When this happens the complete blockage and spasm often relaxes to some degree and air should be able to start moving in and out of the lungs once again. If the patient is not breathing, then some assistance for their ventilation may be needed. Continual BLS assessments should continue.

In the event of an injury the assessment and care of the airway takes precedence over the injury, as without an open airway, death will occur, however if the injury is made worse the patient may not necessarily die. All unconscious patients should be handled with care as to not make any injury worse. Care should be taken to the spine ensuring that no bending or twisting occurs where possible. If possible when moving the patient get someone to support the neck, however this should not delay the movement significantly as an airway assessment must take priority.

The patient should be left on their back when assessing their airway and breathing, apart from submersion injuries where the airway may be filled with water, blood and / or vomitus.

Loose dentures should be removed, however well fitting ones should be left in place, as they may help with obtaining a seal with any bag - mask ventilation device.

If, when opening the mouth, a foreign object is found in the mouth that is easily reachable then use your index finger to scoop it out. If the object is too deep to easily reach then the advice is to leave it as it may go further into the airway and become even more difficult to retrieve later. If the airway is full of fluid / vomit, then turning the patient onto their side to expel it is reasonable. After turning the patient onto their side, a reassessment of their responsiveness and / or breathing should occur and further BLS may be indicated.

After removing any foreign object and / or blood, secretions or other fluid the patient may start breathing spontaneously. If this is the case, then leave the patient on their side in the "recovery position" and await help from trained personnel. Constant patient review and assessment should be undertaken, as it is possible for the patient to require further BLS.

If the adult or child is unresponsive then a "head tilt / chin lift" is recognised as being reasonable[5] if the rescuer is only going to provide chest compressions. There is insufficient evidence to actually recommend that this manoeuvre be carried out when only compressions are provided, but expert opinion recognises that it is likely to be beneficial. In the unconscious patient where full rescue breaths and compressions are to be given by the rescuer then an open airway by means of head tilt/chin lift is recommended.

A head tilt/chin lift is provided by placing one hand on the forehead of the victim and supporting the chin with the rescuer's other hand, gently tilt the head back. Do not apply any significant force as harm may be the result.

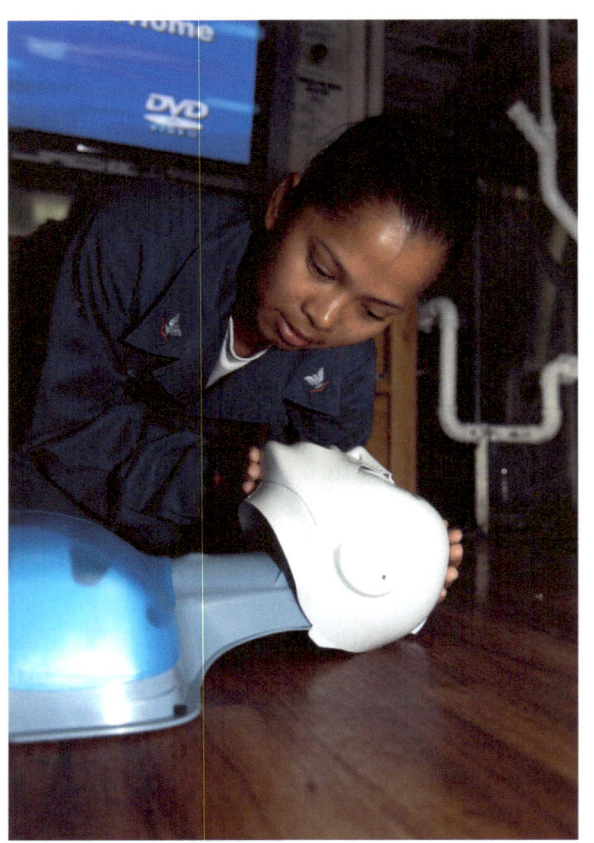

With regards to children and infants: Children (ages 1 - 8 years old) are managed as per adults with regards to airway position[7], however infants (less than 1 year old) are different. Their airway has anatomical differences from adults. Their airways are narrower and as such they can occlude or block easily by using a head tilt / chin lift. As such they are best managed in a neutral position without tilting their head. Having the infants positioned in this way often opens the airway enough, however it is expert opinion that if this does not open the airway sufficiently, then the head may be tilted back very gently is slightly[7][8].

An airway obstruction can be due to several reasons, for example:

- The airway may occlude due to airway muscle relaxation which may be due to unconsciousness.

- There may be a foreign body present which is blocking the airway.

- There may be some form of airway trauma which has caused occlusion of the airway.

- Finally a severe allergic reaction may give cause to an anaphylactic reaction, which due to swelling may close and obstruct the airway.

The use of oropharyngeal airway adjuncts should be only used for the unconscious patients without a gag reflex, as inappropriate use may cause vomiting leading to aspiration.

The use of nasopharyngeal airways has been successfully used for years, however their beneficial use during CPR has not been established by an clinical trials. There have been reports of airway bleeding or other nasal trauma and inter cranial placement when they were placed into patients with basal skull fractures[9]. This is why their use is contraindicated in the presence of a basal skull fracture.

B: Breathing

An obstruction may be partial or complete and may occur immediately, or progress over a period of time. It is therefore essential to keep the patient closely observed throughout the episode. The patient may display paradoxical breathing, where the abdomen rises and the chest sinks and vice-versa. There may also be signs of indentation between the ribs and collar-bones during an attempted inspiration.

Breathing may be absent for a number of reasons, for example:

- Central nervous system depression;

- Near-drowning;

- Asphyxiation;

- Paralysis;

- Airway obstruction.

Whilst in the head tilt / chin lift position place your ear near the patients mouth and look down towards their chest. Look for chest rise and fall, listen for breathing and feel for any breath on your cheek / ear coming from their mouth. Do this for a maximum of 10 seconds. If they are not breathing or not breathing normally go straight to chest compressions.

Although chest compressions are the next step, I am going to put the information on rescue breathing here as it fits with this section better.

Rescue breathing can be provided by either using a medical device such as a bag / mask device or a face mask that you can blow into.

Failing the availability of any device to aid giving the breaths, mouth to mouth breaths may be given. As mentioned earlier, if the rescuer does not want to perform mouth to mouth, then chest compressions should continue. Performing chest compressions is thought to draw some air into the lungs by the changes in intra-thoracic pressure caused by the compressions.

If mouth to mouth is the only option available it is provided by ensuring the airway is open, by keeping the victim in the head tilt / chin lift position, kneeling down next to the them and whilst pinching their nose, keep your mouth open as wide as possible and put it over their slightly open mouth and blow to allow the chest to rise. Try not to over inflate the chest, as this may encourage stomach inflation and possible vomiting / aspiration. Provide the victim's inhalation for 1 second per breath.

Should the chest not rise then this may be due to either an obstruction, not enough air being blown into the victim's lungs or an inadequate seal around the victim's mouth when providing rescue breaths.

With regards to infants it may be more preferable, due to their size, to perform mouth and nose rescue breathing. This is performed by opening the rescuer's mouth as wide as possible and seal it around the victim's mouth and nose. In some cases when the mouth is clamped close mouth to nose breaths may be required. For this technique the rescuer simply seals their mouth over the victim's nose and gives them small rescue breaths. Be aware, however, that in the case of mouth to nose breathing a leak may occur if the victim's mouth is even slightly open. This may stop the chest from rising and subsequently the victim will not receive the necessary life saving breaths. Remember that a paediatric patient has much smaller lungs and a volume of about 6 mls/Kg should be aimed for. Obviously this cannot be accurately measured when providing BLS, so careful observation should be made upon the paediatric's chest for a rise to indicate a satisfactory breath volume.

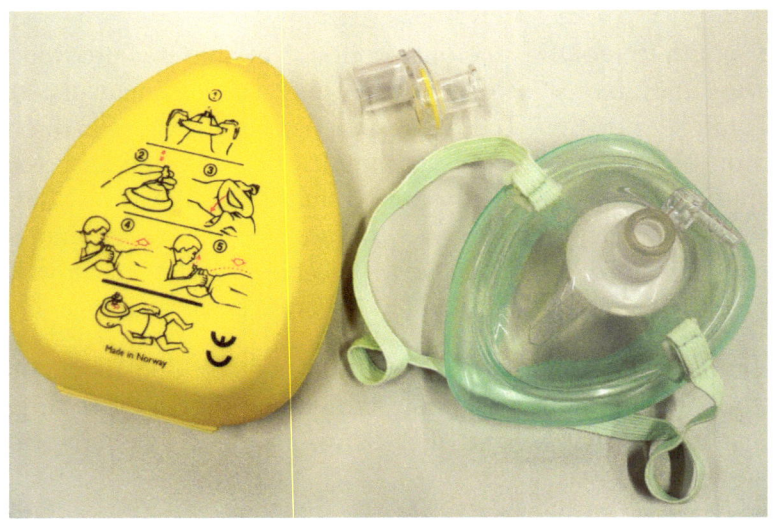

The idea of mouth to mouth, mouth to nose and mouth and nose rescue breathing can cause people to feel at risk of transmission of diseases. In theory this is possible and devices are available to mitigate this risk, such as masks and other barriers. This said, no human studies have shown that a barrier does reduce any transmission[4]. Several reports advise that these barriers be used to reduce the potential risk and there are three studies that have shown a proven reduction in risk of transmission of bacteria in a laboratory environment[4]. There have been reports of transmission of bacteria since 1744 when mouth to mouth ventilation was established. These bacteria included tuberculosis (1 case), Neisseria meningitidis (4 cases), Herpes simplex (2 cases), Helicobacter pylori (1 case), Shigella sonnei (1 case) and Salmonella infantis (1 case)[10]. There have been no reported cases of hepatitis B, C or HIV transmission from mouth to mouth resuscitation[10].

C: Circulation

When an unresponsive patient is not breathing or not breathing normally chest compressions are recommended. There is no need for a pulse check as it is believed following expert opinion that lay persons' assessment of a presence of a pulse is often inaccurate and it can often delay commencing chest compressions. Chest compressions are given by clasping your hands together, one on top of the other and placing one heel of the hand on the lower half of the sternum (breastbone) and compressing 1/3 of the depth of the chest at a rate of 100 compressions per minute. Compress the chest for 30 compressions and then provide 2 breaths (if rescue breaths are to be given by a rescuer).

In infants it may be more preferable to provide a two thumb technique for the compressions due to the victim's size. Some larger children may suit a one handed chest compression technique.

There are significant risks of rib and sternal fractures being sustained by the victim, however this risk is outweighed by the benefit of providing the CPR. Providing the CPR may cause fractures...... not providing it is likely to eventuate death.

D: Defibrillation

Defibrillation used to only be provided in the realm of advanced life support, however it is now a common place in basic life support due to the life saving advances of automated external defibrillators (AED's). The premise is simple with these devices: Switch them on and follow the prompts.

The majority of adults have a cardiac arrest due to a couple of rhythms (ventricular fibrillation and ventricular tachycardia), both of which are treatable with defibrillation. These rhythms also have the greatest chance of reversibility compared to other cardiac arrest rhythms.

As these shockable rhythms are the most common adult arrest rhythms and that they have the greatest chance of reversal, defibrillation should be performed, if appropriate, as soon as possible to increase the chances of a return of spontaneous circulation.

Choking

When presented with a choking patient the key to their treatment is how they are coughing. Coughing is the natural way that the human body tries to expel the foreign object. If they are coughing adequately then reassurance and encouragement for them to cough further should be given. If they fail to cough the foreign object out, an ambulance should be called. If they are not coughing strongly enough to expel the item then there are two techniques that are thought to be useful. The use of abdominal thrusts used to be advised, however currently due to evidence of 32 life threatening complications associated with abdominal thrusts this technique is not recommended[5].

If the patient is conscious then 5 back blows should be performed with the heal of the hand making contact in the middle of the back at the level of the shoulder blades. Ideally support the patient's chest with one hand and lean them slightly forward when giving them the back blows. If that fails to dislodge the foreign object, and the patient is still breathing, then giving them 5 chest thrusts is the next option. This is done in the same manner as chest compressions during CPR, but the compressions are sharper and slower. If that fails to dislodge the object and again the patient is still breathing, then return to the back blows. This treatment can be provided in either a sitting or standing position[5]. In the case of infants, it may be more practical to lay them across your knees to perform these treatments. If the object is dislodged after a few back blows or chest thrusts it is not necessary to continue until 5 is completed. At anytime, if the patient stops breathing, then BLS should be commenced and help sought.

Adult Advanced Life Support

Advanced life support (ALS) is essential to provide the necessary critical thinking and care necessary to revert a patient from an arrested state to that of consciousness and potential recovery. This said however, basic life support is the cornerstone of any good resuscitation effort. Without correct and adequate basic life support the chance of a recovery is near impossible. Upon arriving at an arrest it is the ALS trained individual's primary priority to ensure that the basic life support is adequate in terms of chest compression rate, depth, positioning and technique. The ALS trained individual should also ensure that rescue breathing (if provided) is provided effectively. Feedback should be given to the basic life support providers to ensure effectiveness and change roles with the providers where necessary.

Defibrillator Pad Placement

Hopefully the original rescuers have placed defibrillator pads on the patient's chest. The pads should be placed in the following positions:

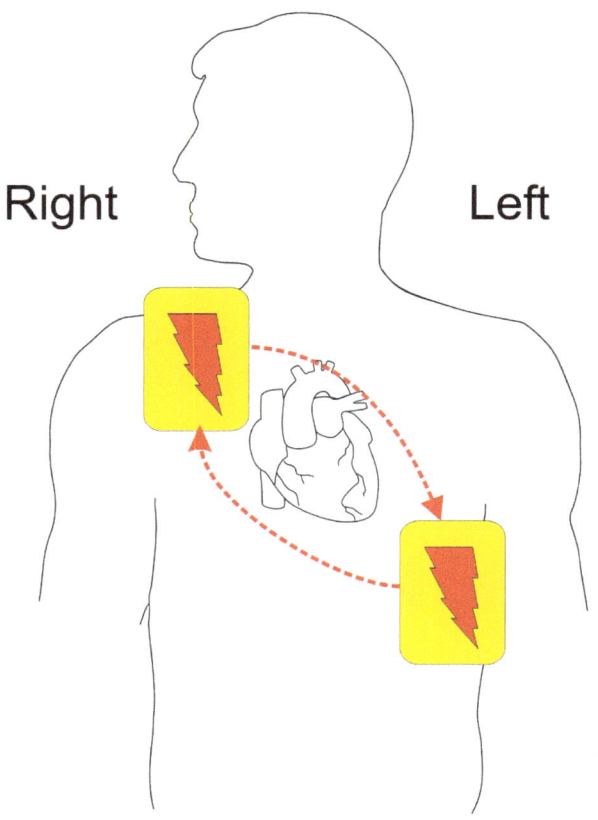

Right   Left

Alternative defibrillator pad placement is known as AP, or anterior - posterior position. In this position the anterior pad is placed on the left apex of the patient's chest over the heart and the posterior pad is placed on the patient's back just behind the heart. This position is a lot less practical as the rescuer needs to roll the victim to place the posterior pad. As such the anterior placement as shown in the prior image is often preferable.

How To Safely And Effectively Defibrillate

A quick observation of the patient's rhythm should be conducted, but to minimise the time when chest compressions are being carried out on the victim it is important to clearly explain to the people performing basic life support what needs to happen.

A good pneumonic through this process is "COACHED". This would be performed as followed. Once the defibrillator pads were applied and whilst chest compressions continue the ALS trained rescuer would clearly instruct other rescuers and follow these prompts:

"**C**hest compressions continue......

Oxygen and everyone else.....

Away..........

Charging the defibrillator.......

Hands off!

Evaluate rhythm

Defibrillate or dump the charge"

Shockable Rhythms

During the evaluation stage of the "COACHED" pneumonic the rhythm is assessed. If the patient is in shockable rhythm a 200J (bi-phasic) or 360J (mono-phasic) shock should be administered. If the patient is not in a shockable rhythm, then the charge should be dumped safely and chest compressions continue. Knowing the defibrillator being used is important, as there are a few ways to dump the charge safely on various defibrillators. Some have a dump button, but many defibrillators charge can be disarmed by reducing the joules selected, or changing the mode from defibrillate to monitor. It is imperative that chest compressions do not continue when the defibrillator is fully charged. If gel pads and paddles are being used the paddles should be replaced in the defibrillator and the charge disarmed safely.

It is at this point that knowing the ALS algorithm is imperative, as depending upon the rhythm identified as being shockable or otherwise will direct the care needed. The following image shows the algorithm, which is provided by the Australian Resuscitation Council. The algorithm may vary slightly depending on which country you live in, however the principles should be very similar, as this is evidence based from ILCOR.

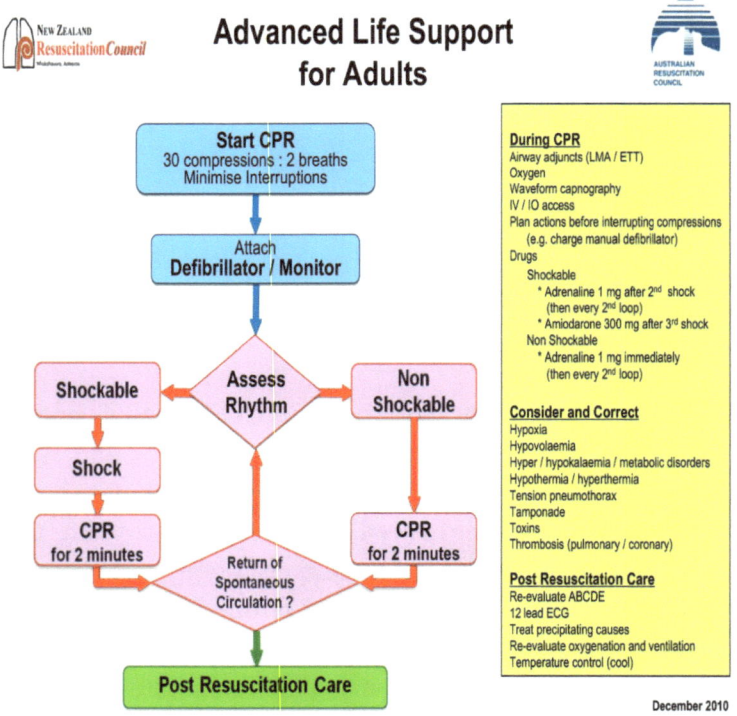

As the algorithm dictates, if the patient was in a shockable rhythm, then they should be defibrillated, as discussed previously. Then 2 minutes of CPR should be performed. At the end of the 2 minutes of CPR if there are no signs of life then another rhythm check should be performed using the "COACHED" pneumonic. Again if the patient is in a shockable rhythm then another 200J (bi-phasic) or 360J (mono-phasic) shock should be administered, followed by another 2 minutes of CPR. It is on commencing this round of CPR that 1mg of adrenaline should be given, prior to another COACHED pneumonic. When the 2 minutes of CPR is nearly complete another COACHED process should be completed and a shock administered if an appropriate rhythm was identified. Following this 3rd shock and during the CPR 300mg of amiodarone can be given. If there is a change in rhythm that is noticed during the 2 minutes of CPR following the shock it is advised to continue CPR, as if there is a return of spontaneous circulation, it is unlikely to be sustained. Therefore a check of pulse should only be done if there are signs of life, or upon a change in heart rhythm which can sustain life when performing a COACHED pneumonic.

Non-Shockable Rhythms

When an adult patient arrests and is not in a shockable rhythm, which is identified when performing a COACHED pneumonic (as previously explained), the defibrillator needs to be safely disarmed, CPR recommenced and 1mg of adrenaline should be administered as soon as possible. CPR should continue for 2 mins, followed by a COACHED and rhythm assessment. If the patient remains in a non-shockable rhythm then again, the defibrillator should be disarmed and CPR recommenced for another 2 minutes. Towards the end of this 2 minutes of CPR another COACHED should be used. If the patient remains in a non-shockable rhythm, another 1mg of IV adrenaline should be given and CPR recommenced immediately.

Severe Bradycardias

Severe bradycardias which have caused the patient to be symptomatic may be treated with atropine, however they may also need to be treated with emergency pacing.

Atropine is still regarded as the first drug of choice in symptomatic brady-arrhythmias, which is given in 500 - 600 mcg doses, repeated every 3 - 5 minutes up to a total of 3mg. Atropine, however, in the paediatric population is only recommended in patients with vagal stimulation or cholinergic drug toxicity[10].

Once 3mg of atropine is given a low dose of adrenaline / epinephrine may be considered with doses in the range of 2 - 10 mcg/min. This is given to aim for a suitable heart rate that sustains a mean arterial blood pressure of 70 mmHg.

Pacing can be provided using the defibrillator if it has a pacing mode. This can be achieved by selecting the pacing mode and turning the pacing rate to something reasonable such as 60 - 80 beats per minute and then turn the output up on the pacing unit until a capture of a QRS is seen. Once this has been achieved it is important to reassess the patient with regards to airway, breathing and circulation.

External pacing is uncomfortable and the patient will need some form of sedation +/- analgesia to tolerate it until some more sustaining form of pacing can be sourced, which may or may not be appropriate. Temporary trans-venous pacing is the optimal choice in the short term.

Complete or third degree heart blocks also often need urgent pacing, however unless they are extremely symptomatic (pre-arrest) they often can receive primary transvenous pacing without any major issue. This said however it does not take away the benefit of a thorough patient assessment and clinical judgement. Atropine is unlikely to be beneficial in these patients due to its pharmokenetics of stimulating the AV node. Complete or third degree heart block is the dissociation between the atria and ventricles. Stimulating the AV node in this rhythm does not help the rhythm.

Severe tachyarrhythmias

If the patient is not rapidly deteriorating the regularity of the patient's rhythm needs to be established.

If the rhythm is regular and narrow and if vagal manoeuvres are not successful, then a rapid bolus 6mg dose of adenosine may be useful, followed by a 12mg dose if that is unsuccessful. Should the 12mg dose not revert the patient to a sinus rhythm then expert opinion should be sought and atrial flutter may be considered, which may require the use of beta blockers to control the heart rate. If the adenosine did revert the patient to a sinus rhythm then consideration should be made regarding the need for anti-arhythmic prophylaxis.

Tachyarrhythmias which are irregular and narrow are likely to be atrial fibrillation in origin and if the patient is stable consideration needs to be made regarding the use of an IV beta blocker, digoxin to control the heart rate +/- amiodarone infusion.

Stable patients showing a regular broad complex tachycardia are to be treated as if they are in a ventricular tachycardia and a 300mg amiodarone bolus over 20 - 30 minutes followed by a 900mg over 24 hours may be considered. Should the patient have previous confirmed SVT with a bundle branch block then a 6mg dose of adenosine, followed by a 12mg dose may be indicated.

For stable patients who have a broad complex and irregular rhythm, expert opinion should be sought, as the rhythm could be an atrial fibrillation with a bundle branch block, pre-excitation atrial fibrillation, or a polymorphic ventricular tachycardia / torsades des points. Should the patient's rhythm be diagnosed as an atrtial fibrillation with a bundle branch block, then they should be treated as a narrow complex atrial fibrillation. If the patient's diagnosed with a pre-excitation atrial fibrillation then amiodarone may be considered. In the presence of a polymorphic ventricular tachycardia or torsades des points, then a 5mmols of magnesium over 10 minutes may be considered, which may be repeated once and accompanied with an infusion of 20mmols over 4 hours[11].

Tachycardias which cause the patient to be symptomatic and rapidly deteriorating may need cardioversion. This needs to be given by using the "Sync" button which will deliver the shock on the R wave to revert the rhythm. If the "Sync" button is not pressed it is possible to put the patient into another rhythm such as VF, VT or asystole. It is not abnormal to start with 100J shock and then goto 150J and finally 200J. Sedation may be needed for the cardioversion, as it would be uncomfortable. If these shocks do not revert the patient then a 300mg dose of amiodarone may be indicated.

Once 3 cardioversions are attempted then a 300mg dose followed by 900mg of amiodarone over 24 hours may be considered in the absence of polymorphic ventricular tachycardia or torsades des points. Patients in polymorphic ventricular tachycardia or torsades des points should be treated with 5 mmols of magnesium given over 10 minutes, which may be repeated once and accompanied with an infusion of 20mmols over 4 hours[11].

Broad complex tachycardias should be treated as ventricular tachycardia until proven otherwise. It is true that a broad complex tachycardia could be an SVT with a bundle branch block or some other form of aberrant conduction, however treating a VT as an SVT has worse outcomes than treating an SVT as a VT[11].

Causes Of Arrests

The reason why a patient has arrested need to be identified as soon as the person is found in an arrested state. The easiest way of remembering reasons for cardiac arrest are by referring to "4 H's and 4 T's". They are as follows:

- **H**ypoxia

- **H**ypo / **H**yperthermia

- **H**yperkalaemia / **H**ypokalaemia

- **H**ypovolaemia

- **T**amponade

- **T**ension pneumothorax

- **T**oxins / Poisons / Drugs

- **T**hrombotic embolus

How To Treat The Causes

Hypoxia

Hypoxic arrests are treated by ensuring the patient receives 100% oxygen during the cardiac arrest. An artificial airway may be needed to provide additional positive pressure ventilatory support with the potential benefits of PEEP (Positive End Expiratory Pressure). An artificial airway is considered by many to be more superior compared to bag mask ventilation, as it provides some form of airway protection, reduced risk of gastric hyperinflation and potential aspiration. There is not any evidence however to support endotracheal intubation during a cardiac arrest[9]. If the prolonged arrest is due to hypoxia, then providing the patient with an advanced airway may be appropriate. The benefit of an endotracheal intubation, associated with the risk of unrecognised oesophageal intubation, or malplacement need to be considered. The clinician may also not be able to intubate the patient, despite their level of skill, and the patient may suffer damaging hypoxia.

Hypo / Hyperthermia

Hypothermia is often seen in patients who have suffered from exposure. Normally the body remains around 37°C, however hypothermia can occur below 35°C. In this circumstance remove any source of cold, removing wet cold clothes, removing them from the cold environment where possible, where possible also give warm fluids when indicated. People can remain in a cardiac arrest for a long time and there is a saying in critical care, "You cannot be certified as dead until you are warm and dead." Normothermia prior to any cessation of ALS providing measures should be considered.

Hyperthermic patients needs to be cooled to normothermia by applying ice to their body where possible. Moisten the skin by applying cold wet cloths if ice is not available or appropriate due to other ALS activity. The use of rapid infusion of cold saline or ringers solutions have been well demonstrated in the literature[12]. Move the patient also, if possible, out of the direct sunlight into some shaded area.

Hypo / Hyperkalaemia

Potassium is an essential chemical in the body, however a significant imbalance is a reason to arrest and its correction is imperative. In the hypokalaemic state give 5 mmols potassium chloride intravenously and repeat as necessary. Generally intravenous potassium is only given in concentrated forms via a central venous line, however in the arrested patient it is permissible to give it peripherally or through the intraosseous route. Be aware that extravasation may occur through peripheral administration, which may lead to tissue necrosis. This said however, the patient is dead without the drug and the risk of giving the drug peripherally outweighs the risk of possible extravasation. In some situations 5 mmols magnesium is also given when hypokalaemia is present, as a low magnesium often accompanies hypokalaemia. An infusion of 20 mmols over 4 hours may also be indicated upon receiving blood results.

Hyperkalaemia is treated by administering 10 mls of 10% calcium chloride, which is 6.8 mmols. In addition to the calcium, sodium bicarbonate is often given at a dose of 1 mmol / Kg over 2 - 3 minutes. It is then repeated as guided by the arterial blood gas results.

Hypovolaemia

A low circulating volume is a very valid reason for a cardiac arrest. The treatment of such is to give 20 mls / Kg of normal saline. This is repeated as necessary.

Hypovolaemia can occur for many reasons, such as:

- Blood loss with either internal or external haemorrhage.

- Plasma losses due to burns and other wounds discharging fluids

- Excessive sodium excretion or sodium loss due to excessive sweating, vomiting or diarrhoea. The loss of sodium causes an associated loss of intravascular water which needs to be replaced.

- Vasodilation due to a multitude of factors, including trauma, sepsis and medications.

Tamponade

A cardiac tamponade is a situation where bleeding occurs within the pericardial sac. This increase in bleeding causes an increase in pressure exerted on the heart which reduces the contractility and subsequent cardiac output. In times past this situation had very bad outcomes. The outcomes are still not fantastic, but they are a lot better than they used to be. A needle used to be inserted blindly whilst exerting some negative pressure on the syringe. This had its obvious risks. Today this procedure is best performed under ultrasound guidance[13].

Tension pneumothorax

A tension pneumothorax can occur spontaneously, as a result of trauma and also due to positive pressure ventilation. A pneumothorax is a build up of gas in the pleural space. If this leak creates a one way valve or the pressure in the pleura is excessive the pneumothorax will extend and not only compress the affected lung, but it will also begin to compress the non-affected lung. Tracheal deviation may be present accompanied with significant shortness of breath. Immediate treatment of this is to place a large-bore needle mid-clavicular in the second intercostal space of the affected side. A hissing noise should be heard as the build up of air is released out of the needle. When this diagnosis has been made a chest drain should be inserted.

Toxins / Poisons / Drugs

When presented with poisoning or toxins it is important to make an assessment as to what has been ingested. If it is an overdose of an opiate then naloxone can be given. The doses used can be variable, ranging from 100 mcg to 2 mg (see drugs section). Tricyclic antidepressant overdosing is best treated with sodium bicarbonate due to the metabolic acidosis and other supportive measures for arrhythmia's. Beta blocker overdose can be treated with glucagon, however high dose insulin therapy can also be considered. Glucagon is the drug of choice for many as it is positively inotropic, chronotropic and dromotropic. For a thorough and concise strategy in treating any poisoning or overdoses the local poisoning unit or toxicologist should be consulted.

Thrombo-embolisms

A thrombotic embolus that has caused a cardiac arrest is likely to be either that of a myocardial, pulmonary or cerebral in origin. If it is indeed an embolus then treatment with fibrinolytic therapy may be indicated. Being in an cardiac arrest, needing CPR is not a contraindication to being thrombolysed. If fibrinolytic therapy is given then it is suggested to continue CPR for another 30 minutes to allow for effect of the therapy[14].

Return Of Spontaneous Circulation

Normally during effective CPR it will not be possible to easily notice a change in rhythm confidently and a pause in CPR should only occur during a "COACHED" event. If for some reason a change in rhythm is noticed during the 2 minutes of CPR it is recommended that compressions continue until the end of the 2 minutes. Equally, if the patient is shocked out of a shockable rhythm into a perfusable rhythm it is recommended that compressions continue for another 2 minutes. The reason for this is that if perfusion and a pulse is felt immediately post a shock or during the 2 minutes of compressions the pulse is not likely to be sustained. Therefore we should only be checking for a pulse in the presence of a perfusable rhythm after 2 minutes of compressions during a COACHED event[15].

Return of spontaneous circulation can be seen in many ways, however the international advanced life support community are advocating the use of end tidal carbon dioxide capnography to detect both adequate ventilation, but it also helps to identify a return of spontaneous circulation. The theory is that when the carbon dioxide level starts to rise towards normal limits it is indicative of the heart beating again and as such removing carbon dioxide from the blood.

Return of spontaneous circulation is obviously identified if the patient makes any form of purposeful movement.

In the event of signs of return of spontaneous circulation a pulse check should be performed, followed by ABCDE checks and post-resuscitation care, as discussed next.

Post Resuscitation Care

The post resuscitation care is arguably just as important as the advanced life support itself, as without proper post resuscitation care the patient is unlikely to have a very good outcome and is at an increased risk of going into another cardiac arrest.

The assessment and treatment of any abnormalities in the airway, breathing or circulation of the patient is essential. This may include continuation of mechanical ventilation +/- inotropes / vasopressors as required. The aim of preventing a hypoxic brain injury, myocardial depression, ischaemia and infarct are very important along with reducing risk of other end organ dysfunction. Maintaining cerebral perfusion through an adequate mean arterial pressure of above 60mmHg, treating reversible cardiac arrhythmias, along with the continual treatment of the initial cardiac arrest. Once the ABC has been addressed it is essential to treat the D & E of disability and environment. If the patient was neurologically intact prior to the arrest and they are not now, then an induced hypothermia may be indicated, aiming for a core temperature of 32 - 34°C for 12 - 24 hours[12]. Blood sugar should also be monitored and kept within normal limits[12].

The patient may need to be moved to an intensive care unit for post arrest care.

Obtaining Access For Drug Delivery

Getting intravenous access in patients can be a challenge at the best of times, however during a cardiac arrest the task can be even more challenging. Normally in a cardiac arrest scenario intravenous medications are given through a cannula in a large peripheral vein. Ideally veins in the lower limbs should be avoided due to the poor venous return during a cardiac arrest[16].

If normal peripheral access is not achievable then the external jugular vein may be considered, however there is a faster and safer option. An intraosseous device can be used when intravenous access is challenging and access is not achievable within 90 seconds. There are many devices available today for inserting an intraosseous device ranging from the "BIG gun", "FAST 1", "FAST X", "FAST COMBAT", "FAST RESPONDER", "EZ-IO" and standard IO Cook needle. There are many routes to insert an intraosseous device for example:

- 1-2 cm medially and 1 cm proximally to the tibial tuberosity.

- 1-2 cm proximally to the base of the malleolus

- Posterior distal metaphysis of the radium (behind radial pulse)

- Anterior head of the humerus

The great thing about intraosseous insertion is that it is quick, easy and has a high probability of correct placement. All drugs can be infused into the device which permeates the bone marrow. & the doses are the same as those given through IV administration. If fluid boluses are needed, then need to be put in under pressure as they will not feed into the bone marrow satisfactorily by gravity alone.

Drugs

Adrenaline or Epinepherine

IV adrenaline can be given every 2nd loop. It is given immediately for a non-shockable rhythm and then every 2nd loop. In a shockable rhythm it is given after the second loop of shocks. The theory behind the drug is that is is going to improve probability of cardiac contraction and it will also improve peripheral arterial smooth muscle constriction and subsequent blood flow to vital organs.

Amiodarone

Amiodarone is given in a refractory VF or VT situation. This is where the shockable rhythm is resistant to cardioverting to a life sustaining rhythm. It is given by diluting 300mg in 10 - 20 mls of 5% dextrose (glucose) and given as a bolus. Ideally this should be flushed with 10 - 20 mls of 5% dextrose to ensure good delivery of the drug to the central circulation. It is mixed with dextrose, as this drug is incompatible with saline and has a high risk of precipitating. Amiodarone is a broad spectrum anti-arrhythmic which may also be used to treat refractory shockable rhythms in an advanced life support situation.

Atropine

Atropine is the first line medication for the treatment of severe bradycardias which cause the patient to become symptomatic. The drug is given intravenously in doses of 500 - 600 mcg and can be repeated every 3 - 5 minutes up to 3 mg[11]. If this fails to revert the bradyarrhythmia, adrenaline can be used in doses of 2 - 10 mcg intravenously[11].

Calcium Chloride

Calcium is needed in the treatment of calcium channel blocker overdose, hyperkalaemia. It is generally given by administering 10mls of 10% calcium chloride which is 6.8 mmols[17].

Lignocaine or Lidocaine

Lignocaine is a sodium channel blocker and is useful when amiodarone is not available or cannot be given. It is given in doses of 1 mg / Kg. Amiodarone should be the first line drug of choice in refractory or recurrent VF/VT as demonstrated by two randomised control trials[17].

Magnesium Sulfate

Magnesium is not just given due to hypomagnesia, but also in hypokalaemic states, as when potassium is low, magnesium is often also low. It is also the treatment of choice in torsade de points, or poly-morphic ventricular tachycardia. This is done by giving a 5 mmols bolus, which can be repeated once, followed by a 20 mmols over 4 hours[18].

Naloxone

Naloxone is the drug used to treat opiate overdose. The drug has not been found to improve survival rates of people in cardio-pulmonary arrest, but it has been seen as useful in the pre-arresting patient[14]. The dose can vary, but doses can range from 100 mcg to 2 mg. 100 mcg may relieve the effects to some small degree, however a large 2 mg dose will completely reverse the effects and cause withdrawal with possible negative risks of harm to both the patient and the clinician[14]. Usually in an arrest scenario 200 - 400 mcg doses are commonly given.

Potassium Chloride

Potassium chloride is used to treat hypokalaemia. This is done by giving 5 mmols intra-venously. It is usually given and preferably given via a central line due to the risks of extravasation, however in an arrest situation giving 5 mmols peripherally is acceptable[18].

Sodium Bicarbonate

Sodium bicarbonate combines with hydrogen ions to form a weak carbonic acid which breaks down to form water and carbon dioxide. The swift use of CPR and effective ventilation often negate the need for this drug and it is not recommended through expert consensus opinion[18].

The use of sodium bicarbonate can be considered for hyperkalaemia, protracted arrests greater than 15 minutes, tricyclic antidepressant overdose, or for a metabolic acidosis. The clinician needs to be aware that the use of sodium bicarbonate will cause an increased intra-cellular acidosis as the additional free carbon dioxide enters the cells. There is also some evidence that sodium bicarbonate mixed with adrenaline or calcium may counteract each other, precipitate or block the IV line. If the drug is needed, the dose required is 1mmol/K, given over 2 - 3 minutes[18].

Bibliography

1.   Koster, R.W., M.R. Sayre, and M.S. Botha, 2010, Part 5: Adult basic life support: 2010 International consensus on cardiopulmonary resuscitation and emergency cardiovascular care science with treatment recommendations. Resuscitation, 81(1): pp. e40 - e70.

2.   Australian Resuscitation Council, 2012, Recognition and First Aid Management of the Unconscious Victim. 2012 11th January 2014]; Available from: http://www.resus.org.au/policy/guidelines/section_3/unconsciousness.htm.

3.   Sasson, C., et al., 2010, Predictors of survival from out-of-hospital cardiac arrest: a systematic review and meta-analysis. Circulation: Cardiovascular Quality and Outcomes, (3): pp. 63-81.

4.   Berg, M.D., et al., 2010, Part 13: Pediatric Basic Life Support : 2010 American Heart Association Guidelines for Cardiopulmonary Resuscitation and Emergency Cardiovascular Care. Circulation, 122(Suppl. 3.): pp. S862–S875.

5.   Soar, J., et al., 2010, Part 12: Education, implementation, and teams: 2010 International Consensus on Cardiopulmonary Resuscitation and Emergency Cardiovascular Care Science with Treatment Recommendations. Resuscitation, 81(1): pp. e288 - e330.

6.   Australian Resuscitation Council, 2012, Managing an Emergency. 2012; Available from: http://www.resus.org.au/policy/guidelines/section_2/priorities_in_an_emergency.htm.

7.   Australian Resuscitation Council, 2010, Guideline 4: Airway. 2010; Available from: http://www.resus.org.au/policy/guidelines/section_4/guideline-4dec10.pdf.

8.   Arend, C.F., 2000, Transmission of Infectious Diseases through Mouth-to-Mouth Ventilation: Evidence-

Based or Emotion-Based Medicine? Arquivos Brasileiros de Cardiologia, 74(1): pp. 86 - 97.

9.   Australian Resuscitation Council, 2010, Equipment and Techniques in Adult Advanced Life Support. 2010; Available from: http://www.resus.org.au/policy/guidelines/section_11/guideline-11-6dec10.pdf.

10.   de Caen, A.R., et al., 2010, Part 10: Paediatric basic and advanced life support: 2010 International Consensus on Cardiopulmonary Resuscitation and Emergency Cardiovascular Care Science with Treatment Recommendations. Resuscitation, 81: pp. e213 - e259.

11.   Australian Resuscitation Council, 2009, Managing Acute Dysrhythmias. 2009; Available from: http://www.resus.org.au/policy/guidelines/section_11/guideline-11-9nov09.pdf.

12.   Australian Resuscitation Council, 2010, Post-resuscitation Therapy in Adult Advanced Life Support. 2010; Available from: http://www.resus.org.au/policy/guidelines/section_11/guideline-11-7dec10.pdf.

13.   Bodson, L., K. Bouferrache, and A. Vieillard-Baron, 2011, Cardiac Tamponade. Current Opinion in Critical Care, 17(5): pp. 416-424.

14.   Australian Resuscitation Council, 2011, Guideline 11.10: Resuscitation In Special Circumstances. 2011 14/06/2013]; Available from: http://www.resus.org.au/policy/guidelines/section_11/guideline-11-10-nov2011.pdf.

15.   Australian Resuscitation Council, 2010, Cardiopulmonary Resuscitation for Advanced Life Support Providers. 2010; Available from: http://www.resus.org.au/policy/guidelines/section_11/guideline-11-1-1dec10.pdf.

16.   australian Resuscitation Council, 2010, Medications in Adut Cardiac Arrest. 2010; Available from: http://www.resus.org.au/policy/guidelines/section_11/guideline-11-5dec10.pdf.

17.   Somberg, J.C., et al., 2002, Intravenous lidocaine versus intravenous amiodarone (in a new aqueous formulation) for incessant ventricular tachycardia. American Journal of Cardiology, 90: pp. 853 - 859.

www.ingramcontent.com/pod-product-compliance
Lightning Source LLC
Chambersburg PA
CBHW040926180526
45159CB00002BA/628